I0767635

Table Of Contents

The Importance of Mental Health in the Golden Years 3

Common Mental Health Challenges for Men Over 60 3

Breaking the Stigma: Addressing Mental Health in Older Men 3

Seeking Help: Resources and Support for Men Over 60 3

Chapter 2: Emotional Well-being in the Golden Years 3

Exploring Emotions: Understanding the Emotional Landscape 3

Managing Stress and Anxiety in Later Life 3

Cultivating Resilience and Emotional Strength 3

Nurturing Relationships and Social Connections.....................3

Chapter 3: Cognitive Health and Aging..............................3

Age-Related Cognitive Changes: What's Normal and What's Not 3

Enhancing Cognitive Function: Mental Exercises and Brain Training 3

Nutrition and Brain Health: Eating for Cognitive Well-being...........3

Managing Chronic Conditions: Impact on Cognitive Health.............3

Chapter 4: Maintaining Physical Health for Optimal Mental Well-being 3

The Mind-Body Connection: How Physical Health Affects Mental Health 3

Exercise and Aging: Tailoring Fitness Routines for Men Over 60 3

Nutrition for Mental Health: Foods that Support Brain Function 3

Sleep and Rest: Importance for Mental Restoration 3

Chapter 5: Coping with Loss and Change...........................3

Grief and Bereavement: Navigating Loss in the Golden Years 3

Retirement and Identity: Adjusting to a New Phase of Life 3

Dealing with Loneliness and Isolation 3

Reinventing Purpose: Finding Meaning in Later Life..................3

Chapter 6: Strategies for Self-Care and Mental Well-being 3

Prioritizing Self-Care: Understanding Your Needs and Boundaries..3

Mindfulness and Meditation: Cultivating Present Moment Awareness 3

Hobbies and Creative Outlets: Nurturing Passion and Joy 3

Seeking Professional Help: Therapy and Counseling Options 3

Chapter 7: Building a Supportive Community 3

The Power of Support: Establishing Meaningful Connections 3

Men's Groups and Support Networks: Finding Camaraderie.............3

Communicating with Loved Ones: Strengthening Relationships 3

Mentoring and Giving Back: Sharing Wisdom and Experience 3

Chapter 8: Embracing Aging with Resilience and Positivity.................3

Embracing Age-Related Changes: Accepting and Adapting 3

Positive Aging: Challenging Ageist Stereotypes and Beliefs 3

Celebrating Life's Milestones: Finding Joy in the Golden Years.......3

Leaving a Legacy: Reflecting on Your Life's Journey 3

Conclusion: Navigating Your Golden Years with Confidence and Mental Well-being..3

Chapter 1: Understanding Men's Mental Health After 60.....................1

Chapter 1: Understanding Men's Mental Health After 60

The Importance of Mental Health in the Golden Years

As men enter their golden years, it becomes increasingly important to prioritize their mental health. While physical health often takes the spotlight, mental well-being is equally significant and can greatly impact overall quality of life. In this subchapter, we will explore the importance of mental health for men over 60 and delve into strategies for maintaining optimal well-being during this stage of life.

One crucial reason to focus on mental health in the golden years is the prevalence of age-related mental health conditions. Depression, anxiety, and cognitive decline are common challenges that men may face as they age. These conditions can significantly impact daily functioning, relationships, and overall happiness. By addressing mental health concerns proactively, men can prevent or manage these conditions effectively, leading to a more fulfilling and enjoyable life.

Moreover, mental health directly affects physical health. Research has shown that individuals with poor mental health are more likely to experience chronic physical conditions such as heart disease, diabetes, and obesity. By taking care of their mental well-being, men over 60 can reduce their risk of developing these conditions and maintain a higher level of physical health.

Another crucial aspect to consider is the impact of social connections on mental health. As men age, significant life changes, such as retirement, loss of loved ones, or becoming empty nesters, can lead to feelings of isolation and loneliness. Strong social connections are essential for maintaining mental well-being, as they provide support, companionship, and a sense of belonging. Engaging in activities and building new friendships can help combat these feelings of loneliness and enhance overall mental health.

In this subchapter, we will also explore various strategies to promote mental health in the golden years. These may include engaging in regular physical activity, adopting healthy lifestyle habits, practicing stress reduction techniques, and seeking professional help when needed. We will provide practical advice and resources tailored specifically for men over 60, ensuring they have the tools to navigate this stage of life with optimal mental well-being.

By prioritizing mental health in the golden years, men can enhance their overall quality of life, maintain physical health, and cultivate meaningful connections. This subchapter will empower men over 60 with the knowledge and strategies to navigate the challenges and embrace the opportunities of this chapter of their lives.

Common Mental Health Challenges for Men Over 60

As men enter their golden years, they may face various mental health challenges that are unique to this stage of life. It is important for men over 60 to be aware of these challenges and take steps to maintain their mental well-being. In this subchapter, we will explore some of the common mental health challenges that men over 60 may encounter and provide strategies for navigating them.

One of the most prevalent mental health challenges for men over 60 is depression. This can be triggered by factors such as retirement, loss of loved ones, or health issues. It is crucial for men to recognize the signs of depression, including feelings of sadness, loss of interest in activities, changes in appetite or sleep patterns, and difficulty concentrating. Seeking professional help and engaging in activities that bring joy and purpose can help combat depression and improve mental well-being.

Another common mental health challenge for men over 60 is anxiety. Retirement, financial concerns, and health issues can contribute to feelings of worry and unease. It is important for men to practice stress management techniques such as deep breathing exercises, mindfulness, and engaging in regular physical activity. Building a strong support network of friends and family can also provide a sense of connection and alleviate anxiety.

Loneliness and social isolation are also prevalent challenges for men over 60. As social circles may shrink due to retirement or loss of loved ones, men may find themselves feeling isolated. Engaging in social activities, joining clubs or community organizations, and maintaining regular contact with friends and family can help combat loneliness and foster a sense of belonging.

Additionally, cognitive decline and memory loss can be concerns for men over 60. Engaging in mentally stimulating activities such as reading, puzzles, and learning new skills can help maintain cognitive function. Regular physical exercise, a healthy diet, and getting enough sleep also contribute to brain health.

In conclusion, men over 60 may face various mental health challenges that are unique to this stage of life. By being aware of these challenges and implementing strategies to maintain mental well-being, men can navigate their golden years with resilience and happiness. Remember, seeking professional help and building a support network are essential steps in addressing mental health concerns.

Breaking the Stigma: Addressing Mental Health in Older Men

As men age, their mental health can face unique challenges. However, discussing these issues openly is often stigmatized, leading many older men to suffer in silence. In this subchapter, we aim to break the stigma surrounding mental health in older men and provide guidance on how to address these concerns.

For men over 60, mental health becomes increasingly important as they navigate the golden years. Retirement, loss of loved ones, and changes in physical health can all contribute to feelings of isolation, depression, and anxiety. Unfortunately, societal expectations often discourage men from seeking help, perpetuating the misconception that admitting to mental health struggles is a sign of weakness.

It is crucial to recognize that mental health is just as important as physical health. By addressing mental health concerns head-on, older men can improve their overall well-being and quality of life. This subchapter will provide strategies and resources to help men over 60 navigate their mental health journey.

We will explore various topics, including coping mechanisms for common mental health challenges, fostering social connections, and seeking professional help when necessary. Through personal stories and expert advice, readers will gain a better understanding of their own mental health and learn to recognize the signs that indicate the need for support.

Additionally, we will delve into the importance of self-care and maintaining a healthy lifestyle. Physical activity, proper nutrition, and engaging in hobbies can all contribute to positive mental well-being. By encouraging menover 60 to prioritize self-care, this subchapter aims to empower them to take charge of their mental health.

Breaking the stigma surrounding mental health in older men is crucial for their well-being. By encouraging open conversations, providing valuable resources, and offering practical strategies, this subchapter will equip men over 60 with the tools they need to navigate their mental health journey. Together, we can create a society where mental health is prioritized, and no one feels ashamed or isolated due to their struggles.

Seeking Help: Resources and Support for Men Over 60

As men age, they often face unique challenges that can impact their mental health. It is crucial for men over 60 to prioritize their mental well-being, as it can significantly influence their overall quality of life. Recognizing the importance of seeking help and finding appropriate resources and support is a vital step towards maintaining mental wellness during the golden years.

One of the first resources to consider is professional help. Mental health professionals, such as therapists or psychologists, are trained to address the specific concerns faced by older men. They can provide a safe space to discuss feelings of loneliness, anxiety, depression, or any other mental health issues. These professionals can also offer guidance on coping strategies and provide personalized treatment plans tailored to each individual's needs.

Joining support groups can also be tremendously beneficial. Connecting with other men who are going through similar experiences can create a sense of camaraderie and understanding. These groups often offer a platform for sharing stories, discussing challenges, and providing mutual support. Local community centers, religious organizations, or online platforms can be excellent places to find such groups.

Technology has made accessing mental health resources easier than ever. Numerous websites and apps offer mental health information, self-help tools, and even virtual therapy sessions. These resources are convenient and can be accessed from the comfort of one's home. They can provide valuable insights, coping strategies, and a sense of empowerment to men over 60 who may not feel comfortable seeking help through traditional means.

Additionally, it is essential to recognize the importance of maintaining physical health. Regular exercise, a balanced diet, and sufficient sleep contribute to overall well-being and can positively impact mental health. Engaging in activities that bring joy, such as hobbies, volunteering, or spending time with loved ones, can also promote mental wellness and provide a sense of purpose.

In conclusion, seeking help and accessing appropriate resources and support is crucial for men over 60 to maintain their mental health during the golden years. Professional help, support groups, online resources, and personal lifestyle choices all play significant roles in promoting mental well-being. By actively seeking help and utilizing the available resources, men over 60 can navigate the unique challenges they may face and enjoy a fulfilling and emotionally healthy life.

Chapter 2: Emotional Well-being in the Golden Years

Exploring Emotions: Understanding the Emotional Landscape

As men embark on the journey of their golden years, it becomes crucial to navigate the emotional landscape that accompanies this new phase of life. Understanding and managing emotions is an integral part of maintaining good mental health. In this subchapter, we will delve deeper into the subject of emotions and discuss their significance for men over 60.

It is essential to acknowledge that emotions are not limited to specific age groups or genders. However, as men age, they may face unique emotional challenges that require careful attention. The purpose of this section is to shed light on these challenges and provide strategies for understanding and addressing them effectively.

One critical aspect of exploring emotions is recognizing that it is normal to experience a wide range of feelings. Men over 60 may encounter emotions such as joy, contentment, sadness, grief, or even anxiety. Understanding that these emotions are a natural part of life can help men embrace their emotional well-being rather than suppress or deny their feelings.

Another important aspect is the impact of societal expectations on men's emotional expression. Throughout their lives, men have often been encouraged to adhere to societal norms that discourage the open expression of emotions. However, in the golden years, breaking free from these expectations is crucial for mental health. It is essential for men to understand that expressing their emotions is not a sign of weakness, but rather a strength that allows for a deeper connection with oneself and others.

Furthermore, exploring emotions involves understanding the interplay between physical and emotional health. Men over 60 may experience age-related physical changes that can have a significant impact on their emotional state. By recognizing this connection, individuals can develop self-care practices that promote both physical and emotional well-being.

To navigate the emotional landscape effectively, men over 60 can benefit from various strategies. These may include seeking support from loved ones, engaging in regular physical activity, practicing mindfulness and relaxation techniques, and considering professional counseling or therapy. The goal is to create an environment that encourages emotional exploration and provides the necessary tools to cope with the challenges that may arise.

In conclusion, understanding the emotional landscape is a vital aspect of men's mental health after 60. By recognizing and embracing their emotions, men can foster a healthier and more fulfilling life. This subchapter serves as a guide to help men over 60 navigate their emotional journey, providing valuable insights and practical strategies to promote emotional well-being in the golden years.

Managing Stress and Anxiety in Later Life

As men enter the golden years of their lives, they may find themselves facing new challenges and experiences that can lead to increased stress and anxiety. It is essential to prioritize mental health during this phase and develop effective strategies to manage these emotions. In this subchapter, we will explore various techniques and tools for managing stress and anxiety in later life, providing valuable insights specifically tailored to men over 60.

1. Recognizing the Signs: It is crucial to understand the signs and symptoms of stress and anxiety. These may include irritability, sleep disturbances, loss of appetite, and feelings of unease. By recognizing these signs, individuals can take proactive steps towards managing their mental health.

2. Physical Activity and Exercise: Engaging in physical activities and regular exercise has been proven to reduce stress and anxiety levels. Whether it's going for a brisk walk, practicing yoga, or participating in a sport, staying physically active can boost mood and promote overall well-being.

3. Mindfulness and Meditation: Incorporating mindfulness and meditation into daily routines can be highly beneficial for managing stress and anxiety. These practices encourage individuals to focus on the present moment, fostering a sense of calm and relaxation.

4. Social Support: Building and maintaining strong social connections is crucial for mental health. Engaging in social activities, joining clubs or organizations, and spending time with loved ones can provide a sense of belonging, reduce loneliness, and alleviate stress.

5. Healthy Lifestyle Choices: Making healthy lifestyle choices, such as eating a balanced diet, getting enough sleep, and limiting alcohol intake, can have a significant impact on mental well-being. Taking care of one's physical health can help manage stress and anxiety.

6. Seeking Professional Help: If stress and anxiety become overwhelming, seeking support from mental health professionals is essential. Therapists and counselors can provide guidance, offer coping strategies, and create personalized treatment plans to address specific concerns.

7. Embracing Hobbies and Interests: Engaging in hobbies and interests that bring joy and fulfillment can significantly reduce stress levels. Whether it's gardening, painting, playing a musical instrument, or learning a new skill, pursuing passions can offer a sense of purpose and relaxation.

By implementing these strategies, men over 60 can effectively manage stress and anxiety, leading to improved mental well-being during their golden years. Prioritizing mental health and adopting healthy coping mechanisms will enable them to navigate this stage of life with grace and resilience, fostering a sense of fulfillment and happiness.

Cultivating Resilience and Emotional Strength

As men enter their golden years, they may find themselves facing a unique set of challenges when it comes to mental health. Navigating the ups and downs of life after 60 can sometimes feel overwhelming, but it is essential to remember that cultivating resilience and emotional strength can greatly contribute to maintaining overall well-being.

Resilience is the ability to bounce back from adversity and navigate life's challenges with grace and strength. It is not an innate trait but rather a skill that can be cultivated over time. Men over 60 can benefit greatly from developing resilience as they face various transitions, such as retirement, loss of loved ones, and declining physical health.

One crucial aspect of building resilience is adopting a positive mindset. It's all too easy to dwell on the negative aspects of aging, but focusing on the positive can make a significant difference in mental health. Embracing gratitude for the experiences and accomplishments of the past, as well as finding joy and purpose in the present moment, can help men over 60 maintain a resilient mindset.

Emotional strength is another vital aspect of men's mental health after 60. It involves developing the skills to manage and express emotions effectively. Society often expects men to be stoic and unemotional, but suppressing emotions can be detrimental to mental well-being. It is essential to understand that it is perfectly acceptable and healthy to acknowledge and express emotions.

Practicing self-care is a valuable tool in building emotional strength. Engaging in activities that bring joy, such as hobbies, exercise, or spending time with loved ones, can help men over 60 experience a range of positive emotions. Additionally, seeking support from friends, family, or professional therapists can provide a safe space for emotional expression and processing.

Cultivating resilience and emotional strength in men over 60 is not a solitary endeavor. Building a strong support network is crucial. Surrounding oneself with individuals who understand and empathize with the unique challenges of aging can provide a sense of belonging and solidarity. Joining groups or organizations focused on men's mental health after 60 can create opportunities for connection and mutual support.

In conclusion, cultivating resilience and emotional strength is essential for men over 60 to navigate the challenges and transitions that come with aging. By adopting a positive mindset, practicing self-care, and building a strong support network, men can enhance their mental well-being and enjoy fulfilling golden years. Remember, it's never too late to develop these skills and create a brighter future for oneself.

Nurturing Relationships and Social Connections

Building and maintaining strong relationships is an essential aspect of overall well-being, especially as we navigate the golden years of life. For men over 60, nurturing relationships and social connections becomes even more crucial, particularly in the context of mental health. In this chapter, we will explore the significance of fostering healthy relationships and social connections as we age, and how these factors contribute to men's mental health after 60.

As we grow older, our social circles may naturally shrink due to various reasons like retirement, loss of loved ones, or physical limitations.

However, it is vital to recognize the importance of staying socially active and connected. Engaging with friends, family, and even joining social groups or clubs can have a profound impact on mental well-being. Meaningful relationships provide emotional support, a sense of belonging, and can help combat feelings of loneliness or isolation that are common among older adults.

To nurture relationships, it is crucial to prioritize effective communication. Open and honest conversations with loved ones can help address any unresolved conflicts, strengthen bonds, and foster understanding. Active listening and empathy play a significant role in building deeper connections with others, allowing for more meaningful and satisfying relationships.

Additionally, it is essential to seek out new social connections to expand one's social network. Joining community groups, volunteering, or participating in hobbies and activities can introduce individuals to like-minded individuals and create opportunities for new friendships. Engaging in group activities can also provide a sense of purpose, increase self-esteem, and enhance overall mental well-being.

Technology can also play a valuable role in nurturing relationships and maintaining social connections. Learning to use smartphones, video calling platforms, and social media can help bridge the gap between physical distances and allow for regular communication with family and friends. It is never too late to explore and embrace new technologies that can keep us connected in this digital age.

In conclusion, nurturing relationships and social connections are vital components of men's mental health after 60. By actively engaging with loved ones, seeking out new social connections, and utilizing technology, men can combat feelings of loneliness, build strong support systems, and enhance their overall well-being. Remember, it's never too late to invest in relationships and create a fulfilling social life, even during the golden years.

Chapter 3: Cognitive Health and Aging

Age-Related Cognitive Changes: What's Normal and What's Not

As we journey through the golden years of life, it's natural to experience certain changes in our cognitive abilities. While some decline in mental sharpness is considered normal with age, it's essential to distinguish between typical age-related cognitive changes and those that may indicate a more serious underlying condition. In this subchapter, we will explore the topic of cognitive changes in men over 60, helping you understand what is normal and what may require further attention.

Normal age-related cognitive changes often include mild forgetfulness, such as occasionally misplacing items or forgetting names momentarily. It's not uncommon to experience a slower processing speed or find it more challenging to multitask compared to your younger years. These changes are usually a result of natural brain aging and do not significantly impact daily functioning or independence.

However, it is crucial to be aware of certain signs that may indicate more than just typical age-related changes. Persistent and worsening memory loss that disrupts daily life, difficulty completing familiar tasks, confusion with time or place, or struggles with problem-solving and decision-making could be warning signs of cognitive impairment or even dementia. If you or a loved one experience these symptoms, it's vital to seek professional evaluation and support.

To maintain optimal cognitive health during the golden years, there are various strategies you can adopt. Regular physical exercise, such as walking or swimming, has been shown to improve cognitive function and reduce the risk of cognitive decline. Engaging in mentally stimulating activities, such as puzzles, reading, or learning a new skill, can also help keep your brain active and agile.

Additionally, maintaining a healthy lifestyle by eating a balanced diet, getting sufficient sleep, managing stress, and staying socially connected can positively impact cognitive well-being. It's important to remember that mental health and cognitive function are interconnected, so prioritizing your emotional well-being is equally essential.

In conclusion, understanding the distinction between normal age-related cognitive changes and those that may require further attention is crucial for men over 60. While some decline in cognitive abilities is expected, it's essential to recognize warning signs that may indicate a more serious condition. By adopting healthy lifestyle habits and staying mentally engaged, you can promote your cognitive well-being and navigate the golden years with confidence and clarity.

Enhancing Cognitive Function: Mental Exercises and Brain Training

As men enter their golden years, it is crucial to prioritize their mental health and well-being. Cognitive function, which includes memory, attention, and problem-solving skills, may decline with age. However, there are various ways to enhance cognitive function and maintain a sharp mind throughout the years. One effective approach is engaging in mental exercises and brain training.

Mental exercises are activities that challenge the brain and stimulate cognitive abilities. These exercises can be as simple as solving puzzles, crosswords, or Sudoku. These activities force the brain to think critically, enhancing memory, concentration, and problem-solving skills. Additionally, reading books, learning new skills, and engaging in stimulating conversations can also contribute to mental exercise. The key is to regularly challenge and stimulate the brain to keep it active and agile.

Brain training, on the other hand, involves using specialized programs or applications designed to improve cognitive function. These programs often focus on specific cognitive skills, such as memory or attention, and use a variety of exercises and games to target those areas. Brain training can be done on personal devices like smartphones or tablets, making it easily accessible for men over 60. Regularly participating in brain training exercises can improve cognitive abilities, helping to maintain mental sharpness and delay cognitive decline.

In addition to mental exercises and brain training, adopting a healthy lifestyle can greatly contribute to men's mental health after 60. Regular exercise, a balanced diet, and sufficient sleep all play a vital role in maintaining cognitive function. Physical activity increases blood flow to the brain, delivering oxygen and nutrients necessary for optimal brain function. A diet rich in fruits, vegetables, whole grains, and lean proteins provides essential nutrients that support brain health. Prioritizing sleep is also important, as it allows the brain to rest and consolidate memories.

In conclusion, enhancing cognitive function is crucial for men over 60 to maintain mental sharpness and overall well-being. Engaging in mental exercises and brain training can stimulate cognitive abilities, improving memory, attention, and problem-solving skills. Additionally, adopting a healthy lifestyle that includes regular exercise, a balanced diet, and sufficient sleep further supports cognitive function. By incorporating these strategies into their daily lives, men over 60 can navigate their golden years with a sharper mind and improved mental health.

Nutrition and Brain Health: Eating for Cognitive Well-being

As men age, it becomes increasingly important to prioritize mental health and cognitive well-being. The golden years can bring about various challenges, including changes in brain function and an increased risk of cognitive decline. However, by making conscious choices about nutrition, men over 60 can support their brain health and maintain mental clarity.

A healthy diet plays a crucial role in promoting cognitive well-being. Research suggests that certain nutrients can enhance brain function and protect against age-related cognitive decline. Incorporating these nutrients into your daily meals can make a significant difference in maintaining mental sharpness.

First and foremost, omega-3 fatty acids are essential for brain health. Found in fatty fish like salmon, mackerel, and sardines, these healthy fats have been linked to improved cognitive function and a reduced risk of dementia. If you're not a fan of seafood, you can obtain omega-3s from plant-based sources such as flaxseeds, chia seeds, and walnuts.

Antioxidant-rich foods are also crucial for protecting the brain from oxidative stress and inflammation. Blueberries, spinach, kale, and other colorful fruits and vegetables are excellent sources of antioxidants. These nutrients have been shown to support memory, attention, and overall brain health.

By adopting a brain-healthy diet and making conscious choices about nutrition, men over 60 can support their mental well-being. Remember to consult with a healthcare professional or nutritionist for personalized advice and guidance. Navigating the golden years can be a fulfilling and mentally thriving experience with the right approach to nutrition and mental health.

Managing Chronic Conditions: Impact on Cognitive Health

In addition to omega-3s and antioxidants, B vitamins are vital for brain function. They help in the production of neurotransmitters and play a role in maintaining cognitive abilities. Foods like whole grains, leafy greens, eggs, and lean meats are rich in B vitamins and should be included in your diet.

Furthermore, it's important to reduce the consumption of processed foods, sugary drinks, and excessive amounts of alcohol. These unhealthy choices can negatively impact brain health and increase the risk of cognitive decline.

Alongside a nutritious diet, staying hydrated is essential for optimal brain function. Dehydration can cause cognitive problems and affect memory and concentration. Make sure to drink plenty of water throughout the day and limit the intake of sugary beverages.

As men enter their golden years, it becomes increasingly important to prioritize their mental health. One crucial aspect that often goes overlooked is the impact of managing chronic conditions on cognitive health. Chronic conditions such as diabetes, heart disease, and arthritis can not only affect physical health but also have a significant impact on mental well-being.

Research has shown that there is a strong connection between chronic conditions and cognitive decline in older adults. The management of these conditions requires careful consideration and attention to ensure that cognitive health is not compromised. This subchapter aims to explore the relationship between chronic conditions and cognitive health and provide strategies for effectively managing both.

One of the key factors to consider is the role of lifestyle choices in managing chronic conditions and preserving cognitive health. Regular physical exercise, a balanced diet, and adequate sleep are essential components of maintaining overall health. Engaging in regular exercise has been shown to improve cognitive function and reduce the risk of cognitive decline. Incorporating brain-stimulating activities such as puzzles, reading, or learning new skills can also have a positive impact on cognitive health.

Additionally, it is important to adhere to medical treatments prescribed for chronic conditions. Compliance with medication regimens, regular check-ups, and follow-ups with healthcare providers are crucial. Men should also be proactive in managing their conditions by staying informed about the latest research and treatments available.

Furthermore, it is essential to address the emotional and psychological impact of managing chronic conditions. Chronic conditions can often lead to feelings of frustration, anxiety, and depression. Seeking support from loved ones, joining support groups, or consulting with mental health professionals can help alleviate these emotional burdens. Engaging in activities that bring joy and purpose, such as hobbies, volunteering, or spending time with loved ones, can also positively impact mental well-being.

In conclusion, managing chronic conditions is not only crucial for physical health but also has a significant impact on cognitive health. By adopting a holistic approach that encompasses lifestyle choices, adherence to medical treatments, and addressing the emotional aspect, men over 60 can effectively manage their chronic conditions while preserving their cognitive health. It is essential to prioritize mental well-being and seek support when needed, as navigating the golden years can be a fulfilling and rewarding experience when both physical and cognitive health are well-maintained.

Chapter 4: Maintaining Physical Health for Optimal Mental Well-being

The Mind-Body Connection: How Physical Health Affects Mental Health

As we enter our golden years, it becomes increasingly important to prioritize our physical and mental well-being. The mind-body connection plays a crucial role in maintaining good overall health, particularly in the context of men's mental health after 60. In this subchapter, we will explore how physical health can significantly impact mental well-being and offer practical tips for nurturing both aspects of our lives.

Physical exercise is a powerful tool that can improve mental health in various ways. Engaging in regular physical activity, such as walking, swimming, or even gardening, not only keeps our bodies fit but also boosts our mood by releasing endorphins, the feel-good hormones. Exercise has been proven to reduce symptoms of anxiety and depression, enhance cognitive function, and promote better sleep, all of which contribute to improved mental well-being.

Another important aspect of the mind-body connection is nutrition. A balanced diet rich in whole foods, fruits, and vegetables provides essential nutrients that support brain function. Omega-3 fatty acids found in fish, for example, have been linked to reduced risk of cognitive decline and improved mood. Additionally, limiting the intake of processed foods, sugar, and alcohol can prevent mood swings, enhance focus, and reduce inflammation in the body, which can contribute to better mental health.

Regular medical check-ups are crucial for maintaining both physical and mental health. Conditions such as cardiovascular disease, diabetes, and thyroid disorders can have a significant impact on mental well-being. By staying proactive and addressing any potential health concerns early on, we can prevent or manage these conditions and minimize their impact on our mental state.

Furthermore, social connections play a vital role in men's mental health after 60. Engaging in social activities, joining clubs or organizations, and maintaining relationships with loved ones can help combat feelings of loneliness and isolation. Loneliness has been linked to an increased risk of depression and cognitive decline, highlighting the importance of nurturing our social connections.

In conclusion, the mind-body connection is a fundamental aspect of men's mental health after 60. By prioritizing physical health through regular exercise, a balanced diet, and medical check-ups, we can significantly improve our mental well-being. Additionally, fostering social connections and engaging in activities that bring us joy can further enhance our overall happiness and quality of life. Remember, it's never too late to prioritize your mental health and enjoy the golden years to their fullest potential.

Exercise and Aging: Tailoring Fitness Routines for Men Over 60

As we age, it becomes increasingly important to prioritize our physical and mental well-being. Regular exercise becomes even more crucial for maintaining a healthy lifestyle and promoting mental health. In this subchapter, we will explore the various aspects of exercise and aging, with a specific focus on tailoring fitness routines for men over 60.

As men over 60, we have unique needs and considerations when it comes to our fitness routines. It's essential to approach exercise with caution, taking into account any pre-existing medical conditions or physical limitations. Consulting with a healthcare professional before beginning any exercise program is highly recommended.

One key aspect of exercise for men over 60 is the inclusion of cardiovascular activities. Engaging in activities such as brisk walking, swimming, or cycling helps improve heart health, maintain a healthy weight, and reduce the risk of chronic diseases such as heart disease and diabetes.

Strength training is another vital component of a fitness routine for men over 60. Incorporating resistance exercises, such as lifting weights or using resistance bands, helps maintain muscle mass, bone density, and overall strength. Strong muscles also contribute to better balance and stability, reducing the risk of falls and related injuries.

Flexibility and balance exercises are equally important as we age. Yoga, Pilates, and tai chi are excellent options for improving flexibility, balance, and coordination. These activities not only enhance physical health but also contribute to stress reduction and overall mental well-being.

It's important to listen to our bodies and modify exercises accordingly. As men over 60, we may need to adjust the intensity or duration of certain activities. Additionally, incorporating rest days into our fitness routines is essential to avoid overexertion and prevent injuries.

Finding an exercise routine that brings joy and fulfillment is crucial for long-term adherence. Engaging in activities we enjoy, whether it's dancing, golfing, or playing tennis, not only keeps us physically active but also contributes to our mental health and social well-being.

In conclusion, exercise plays a vital role in maintaining men's mental health after 60. By tailoring fitness routines to our unique needs and limitations, we can enjoy the benefits of improved cardiovascular health, strength, flexibility, and balance. Remember to consult with a healthcare professional, listen to your body, and find activities that bring you joy. Embrace this chapter of life, and let exercise be your companion in navigating the golden years.

Nutrition for Mental Health: Foods that Support Brain Function

As men enter their golden years, maintaining optimal mental health becomes increasingly important. The aging process can bring about various changes in brain function, such as memory decline, cognitive impairment, and increased risk of mental health disorders. However, there are ways to support and protect your brain health, and one powerful method is through proper nutrition.

In this subchapter, we will explore the vital role that nutrition plays in maintaining and enhancing men's mental health after 60. We will focus on specific foods that support brain function and promote overall cognitive well-being.

1. Omega-3 Fatty Acids: Including sources like fatty fish (salmon, mackerel), walnuts, and flaxseeds in your diet can provide essential omega-3 fatty acids. These healthy fats have been linked to improved memory, reduced risk of depression, and enhanced brain function.

2. Antioxidant-Rich Foods: Blueberries, strawberries, and dark chocolate are packed with antioxidants that protect brain cells from damage caused by free radicals. Antioxidants also have anti-inflammatory properties that can reduce the risk of cognitive decline and age-related mental health disorders.

3. Leafy Green Vegetables: Spinach, kale, and broccoli are excellent sources of essential nutrients like folate and vitamin K, which have been associated with better cognitive function and decreased risk of age-related mental decline.

4. Whole Grains: Opt for whole grains like brown rice, quinoa, and whole wheat bread instead of refined carbohydrates. These grains release glucose slowly, providing a steady supply of energy for the brain. They also contain fiber, vitamins, and minerals that support brain health.

5. Nuts and Seeds: Almonds, walnuts, and sunflower seeds are rich in vitamin E, which has been linked to a reduced risk of cognitive decline. Additionally, these snacks provide healthy fats, antioxidants, and other nutrients that support brain function.

By incorporating these brain-boosting foods into your diet, you can nourish your brain and potentially reduce the risk of mental health disorders such as depression, anxiety, and cognitive decline. Remember to consult with a healthcare professional before making any significant dietary changes, especially if you have specific health concerns or conditions.

In conclusion, nutrition plays a crucial role in men's mental health after 60. By focusing on foods that support brain function, you can enhance cognitive abilities, reduce the risk of age-related mental decline, and promote overall well-being as you navigate the golden years.

Sleep and Rest: Importance for Mental Restoration

As we age, the importance of sleep and rest becomes increasingly evident. For men over 60, the value of quality sleep cannot be overstated. In this subchapter, we will explore the significance of sleep and rest in promoting mental restoration and overall mental health.

Sleep is not just a state of unconsciousness; it is a vital process that allows the brain to rejuvenate and restore itself. During sleep, the brain consolidates memories, processes emotions, and repairs damaged cells. Without adequate sleep, cognitive functions such as memory, attention, and decision-making can be significantly compromised.

For men over 60, getting enough sleep becomes even more crucial. As we age, our sleep patterns change, and we may find it more challenging to fall asleep and stay asleep throughout the night. This can lead to daytime sleepiness, fatigue, and a decline in overall mental well-being. By prioritizing sleep and rest, men over 60 can enhance their cognitive performance, emotional resilience, and overall mental health.

Not only does sleep play a vital role in mental restoration, but restful activities during waking hours also contribute to mental rejuvenation. Engaging in hobbies, meditation, or simply taking quiet moments to relax can help reduce stress levels and promote a sense of calm and balance. Regular breaks throughout the day can also enhance focus, productivity, and mental clarity.

Furthermore, sleep and rest have a profound impact on mood regulation and emotional well-being. Insufficient sleep can lead to irritability, mood swings, and an increased risk of developing mental health conditions such as depression and anxiety. Prioritizing restful activities and establishing healthy sleep habits can significantly improve mental resilience and emotional stability for men over 60.

To optimize sleep and rest, it is important to establish a consistent sleep schedule, create a sleep-friendly environment, and practice relaxation techniques before bed. Additionally, avoiding stimulants such as caffeine and alcohol close to bedtime can help improve sleep quality.

In conclusion, sleep and rest are essential for mental restoration and overall mental health in men over 60. By prioritizing adequate sleep and engaging in restful activities, men can enhance cognitive function, emotional well-being, and overall quality of life. Embracing healthy sleep habits is a crucial step towards navigating the golden years with optimal mental health.

Chapter 5: Coping with Loss and Change

Grief and Bereavement: Navigating Loss in the Golden Years

Losing a loved one is an inevitable part of life, and as we age, the pain of grief can become more profound. In the golden years, men often face unique challenges when it comes to processing loss and navigating bereavement. This subchapter aims to provide guidance and support to men over 60 as they cope with grief, emphasizing the importance of men's mental health after 60.

Grief is a complex and personal journey, and there is no right or wrong way to grieve. It is crucial for men to understand that their emotions are valid and that seeking help or support is not a sign of weakness but a sign of strength. The first step in navigating grief is acknowledging and accepting the pain. It is essential to give yourself permission to grieve and to express your emotions freely.

As men over 60, it is common to have experienced multiple losses, such as the passing of parents, friends, or even a spouse. Each loss can trigger different emotions and bring up unresolved grief from the past. This subchapter explores various coping mechanisms and strategies to help navigate these feelings effectively.

One important aspect of grief is finding healthy ways to honor and remember loved ones. Creating rituals, such as lighting a candle or visiting a special place, can provide comfort and a sense of connection.

It is also important to maintain a support network of friends and family who can listen and provide a safe space for expressing emotions.

This subchapter also addresses the potential impact of grief on mental health. Men over 60 may be more vulnerable to developing depression or anxiety after experiencing loss. Understanding the signs and symptoms of these conditions, along with the available treatment options, is crucial for maintaining mental well-being.

Additionally, this subchapter emphasizes the benefits of seeking professional help, such as therapy or counseling. Mental health professionals can provide guidance, support, and tools to navigate grief effectively. They can also help identify any underlying issues that may be complicating the grieving process.

In conclusion, grief and bereavement are integral parts of the golden years. This subchapter highlights the importance of men's mental health after 60 and offers practical advice for navigating loss. By acknowledging and accepting grief, finding healthy ways to remember loved ones, and seeking support, men can honor their emotions and move forward with resilience and strength. Remember, you are not alone in this journey, and help is available to support you through the grieving process.

Retirement and Identity: Adjusting to a New Phase of Life

Retirement is a significant milestone in a man's life. After decades of hard work and dedication, the time finally comes to bid farewell to the professional world and embark on a new phase of life. However, this transition can bring about a range of emotions and challenges, making it crucial to address men's mental health after 60.

One of the key aspects to consider during this period is the impact retirement can have on a man's identity. For many, their job has not only provided financial security but has also defined who they are. The titles, responsibilities, and achievements associated with their careers become intertwined with their sense of self. Therefore, when retirement comes, it can leave a void that is difficult to fill.

Adjusting to a new phase of life requires men to redefine their identity. It is essential to explore and discover other aspects of themselves beyond their professional accomplishments. Engaging in hobbies, volunteering, or pursuing new interests can help build a new sense of purpose and fulfillment. This period of life offers an opportunity for men to reflect on their values, passions, and what truly brings them joy.

Moreover, retirement can also bring about a sense of loss and isolation. The daily interactions with colleagues and the structure of the workplace suddenly disappear. Loneliness and feelings of insignificance may arise. It is crucial for men over 60 to proactively seek social connections and support systems. Joining clubs, community organizations, or connecting with old friends can help combat these feelings of isolation and foster a sense of belonging.

Additionally, maintaining a healthy lifestyle is vital for men's mental health after 60. Regular exercise, a balanced diet, and sufficient sleep can positively impact mood and overall well-being. Engaging in physical activities like walking, swimming, or yoga can not only improve physical health but also contribute to a positive mental state.

In conclusion, retirement represents a significant life transition that requires men over 60 to adjust and redefine their identity. By exploring new interests, seeking social connections, and maintaining a healthy lifestyle, men can navigate this new phase of life with a sense of purpose, fulfillment, and improved mental health.

Dealing with Loneliness and Isolation

Loneliness and isolation can be common challenges that men face as they navigate the golden years of their lives. After a lifetime of work, family responsibilities, and social interactions, the transition into retirement and the loss of loved ones can leave many men feeling disconnected and alone. However, it's important to remember that you are not alone in these feelings, and there are strategies you can employ to maintain your mental well-being and find fulfillment in this stage of life.

One of the first steps to combatting loneliness is acknowledging and accepting your feelings. It is perfectly normal to experience a sense of loss and isolation during this period. By recognizing these emotions, you can begin to address them head-on. It may be helpful to seek support from friends, family, or even professional counselors who can provide guidance and understanding.

Building and maintaining social connections is crucial for combating loneliness. Seek out opportunities to engage with others who share similar interests or hobbies. Joining clubs, community organizations, or volunteering can help you meet new people and establish meaningful connections. Additionally, reaching out to old friends or family members can help strengthen existing relationships and create a support network.

Embracing technology is another valuable tool in overcoming isolation. With the rise of social media, video calls, and online communities, it has never been easier to connect with others, regardless of physical distance. Engaging in online forums or participating in virtual events and activities can provide a sense of belonging and help alleviate feelings of loneliness.

Taking care of your physical health is also essential for maintaining mental well-being. Regular exercise, a balanced diet, and sufficient sleep can boost your mood and energy levels, allowing you to better cope with feelings of loneliness. Additionally, consider exploring mindfulness practices, such as meditation or yoga, which can help you stay present, reduce stress, and foster a sense of connection within yourself.

Lastly, consider exploring new interests or hobbies that bring you joy and fulfillment. Engaging in activities that you are passionate about can provide a sense of purpose and help combat feelings of isolation. Whether it's learning a new instrument, delving into literature, or taking up a new sport, pursuing your passions can introduce you to new communities and expand your social network.

Remember, dealing with loneliness and isolation is a journey, and it's important to be patient and kind to yourself during this process. By acknowledging your feelings, seeking support, building social connections, embracing technology, taking care of your physical health, and pursuing your passions, you can navigate the golden years with a renewed sense of purpose and fulfillment. You are not alone, and there is a world of opportunities waiting for you to explore.

Reinventing Purpose: Finding Meaning in Later Life

As men enter their golden years, it is common for many to experience a shift in their priorities and a search for deeper meaning in life. Retirement, changes in family dynamics, and the natural process of aging can all contribute to a need to reinvent purpose and find new sources of fulfillment. In this subchapter, we will explore the importance of finding meaning in later life and offer guidance on how to navigate this transformative journey.

One of the key aspects of mental health in older men is having a sense of purpose. Without a clear direction or goals to strive for, it is easy to feel lost or disconnected from life. However, the search for purpose in later life is not about achieving external success or recognition; instead, it is about finding activities and passions that bring joy and a sense of fulfillment.

One way to reinvent purpose is by exploring new hobbies or interests. This could involve learning a musical instrument, taking up painting, or joining a local community group. Engaging in activities that spark curiosity and passion helps maintain mental agility and fosters a sense of accomplishment. These pursuits can also provide opportunities for socialization and connection with others, which are crucial for men's mental health.

Another avenue to consider is giving back to the community. Volunteering can be a rewarding way to contribute to society while also finding personal fulfillment. Whether it's mentoring young adults, working with local charities, or sharing your expertise with others, giving back can provide a sense of purpose and make a positive impact on the lives of others.

Additionally, exploring spirituality and mindfulness can offer a deeper sense of meaning. Engaging in practices such as meditation, yoga, or attending religious services can help cultivate inner peace and provide a framework for understanding the bigger questions in life.

Lastly, it is essential to maintain a healthy mindset and embrace the concept of aging as a new phase filled with opportunities rather than limitations. Accepting the changes that come with age and focusing on self-care, such as regular exercise, a balanced diet, and seeking professional help when needed, are vital components of men's mental health after 60.

In conclusion, reinventing purpose and finding meaning in later life is a transformative journey that requires self-reflection, exploration, and an open mind. By engaging in new activities, giving back to the community, exploring spirituality, and maintaining a positive mindset, men over 60 can navigate their golden years with a sense of purpose, fulfillment, and improved mental health.

Chapter 6: Strategies for Self-Care and Mental Well-being

Prioritizing Self-Care: Understanding Your Needs and Boundaries

As men enter their golden years, taking care of their mental health becomes increasingly important. The aging process can bring about unique challenges and changes, both physically and emotionally. To navigate these years with strength and resilience, it is crucial to prioritize self-care and gain a deeper understanding of your needs and boundaries.

Self-care is not a luxury; it is an essential component of maintaining good mental health. Many men over 60 may have spent their lives prioritizing the needs of others, whether it was their families, careers, or societal expectations. However, now is the time to shift the focus inward and recognize that your own well-being matters.

Understanding your needs is the first step towards effective self-care. Take the time to reflect on what brings you joy, fulfillment, and peace. Whether it's engaging in a favorite hobby, spending time in nature, or connecting with loved ones, identify the activities and experiences that make you feel truly alive. By actively incorporating these elements into your life, you are nurturing your mental well-being and fostering a positive mindset.

However, self-care also involves setting boundaries. As you age, it's important to recognize that you may not have the same energy levels or physical capabilities as before. Be mindful of your limitations and avoid overexerting yourself. This may mean saying no to certain commitments or delegating tasks to others. By establishing clear boundaries, you are prioritizing your own needs and preserving your mental and physical health.

Additionally, seeking support is crucial for men's mental health after 60. Reach out to trusted friends, family members, or professionals who can provide guidance and understanding. Share your concerns, fears, and joys with others who can offer valuable perspectives and support. Surrounding yourself with a strong support network can help alleviate the challenges that come with aging and provide a sense of belonging and connection.

Remember, self-care is an ongoing journey. It requires consistent effort and reflection. As you navigate your golden years, make self-care a priority, understand your needs and boundaries, and embrace the support of those around you. By doing so, you can cultivate a fulfilling and mentally healthy life after 60.

Mindfulness and Meditation: Cultivating Present Moment Awareness

In the fast-paced modern world, it is easy for anyone to get caught up in the hustle and bustle of daily life, especially for men over 60 who are navigating the golden years. However, taking the time to cultivate present moment awareness through mindfulness and meditation can have profound benefits for men's mental health after 60.

Mindfulness is the practice of intentionally paying attention to the present moment without judgment. It involves bringing one's awareness to the sensations, thoughts, and emotions that arise in the here and now. By practicing mindfulness, men over 60 can learn to fully engage with their experiences, rather than getting caught up in regrets about the past or worries about the future.

Meditation is a powerful tool that can complement mindfulness practice. It involves setting aside dedicated time to sit quietly, focus on the breath, and observe the mind and body. Regular meditation can help men over 60 develop a greater sense of calm, clarity, and self-awareness. It can also improve concentration, reduce stress, and promote emotional well-being.

Cultivating present moment awareness through mindfulness and meditation can be particularly beneficial for men's mental health after 60. As they enter this stage of life, they may face unique challenges such as retirement, loss of loved ones, changes in physical health, and a sense of purpose. Mindfulness and meditation can provide a sense of grounding and help men navigate these transitions with greater ease.

Moreover, research has shown that mindfulness and meditation can improve cognitive function, memory, and overall brain health in older adults. These practices can also reduce symptoms of anxiety and depression, increase resilience, and enhance overall life satisfaction. By cultivating present moment awareness, men over 60 can develop a deeper connection with themselves and the world around them, leading to a more fulfilling and meaningful life.

In conclusion, mindfulness and meditation are powerful tools for men's mental health after 60. By dedicating time to cultivate present moment awareness, men can better navigate the challenges of aging and find a greater sense of well-being. Whether through mindfulness practices or meditation, these techniques offer an opportunity for self-reflection, relaxation, and inner growth. Embracing mindfulness and meditation can be a transformative journey that allows men over 60 to fully embrace the golden years with grace and presence.

Hobbies and Creative Outlets: Nurturing Passion and Joy

As men reach their golden years, it is essential to prioritize their mental health and overall well-being. One powerful tool that can contribute to a fulfilling and joyful life is engaging in hobbies and creative outlets. These activities not only provide a sense of purpose and passion but also play a significant role in enhancing mental health.

Hobbies can be as diverse as the men who pursue them. Whether it is woodworking, painting, playing a musical instrument, gardening, or even learning a new language, the key is to find something that brings pleasure and fulfillment. Engaging in such activities provides a sense of accomplishment, boosts self-esteem, and helps combat the feelings of loneliness or isolation that can sometimes accompany the aging process.

One of the greatest benefits of hobbies and creative outlets is the opportunity they provide for personal growth and self-expression. They allow men to explore and develop new skills, which can lead to a renewed sense of purpose and passion. By engaging in activities they enjoy, men can tap into their creativity and gain a fresh perspective on life.

In conclusion, hobbies and creative outlets play a vital role in nurturing passion and joy in men's lives after the age of 60. Engaging in activities that bring pleasure and fulfillment not only enhances mental health but also contributes to personal growth and self-expression. By dedicating time to hobbies, men can find a renewed sense of purpose, combat loneliness, and experience a range of positive emotions. So, let's embrace the power of hobbies and creative outlets and navigate our golden years with enthusiasm and fulfillment.

Seeking Professional Help: Therapy and Counseling Options

Moreover, hobbies and creative outlets provide a much-needed break from the daily routine and the stresses that may come with it. They offer a chance to escape into a world of personal interests and immerse oneself in activities that bring joy and contentment. This time devoted to hobbies can be a form of self-care, allowing men to recharge and rejuvenate their minds.

Furthermore, pursuing hobbies and creative outlets can also foster social connections and a sense of community. Joining clubs or groups centered around shared interests can provide opportunities for social interaction, new friendships, and a sense of belonging. This, in turn, can significantly improve mental health and overall well-being.

As men reach their golden years, it is not uncommon for them to face various mental health challenges. These challenges can range from feelings of loneliness and isolation to depression and anxiety. However, it is crucial to understand that seeking professional help is not a sign of weakness but a courageous step towards better mental well-being. Therapy and counseling options can provide invaluable support and guidance to men over 60 as they navigate the complexities of their mental health.

Therapy and counseling offer a safe and confidential space for individuals to express their thoughts, emotions, and concerns. Trained professionals, such as psychologists, psychiatrists, and licensed therapists, can help men over 60 address and manage their mental health issues effectively. One of the most common types of therapy is talk therapy, where individuals engage in open conversations with their therapists. This type of therapy allows men to explore their feelings, gain insight into their behaviors, and develop coping strategies.

Cognitive-behavioral therapy (CBT) is another approach frequently used in the treatment of mental health issues among older adults. This therapy focuses on identifying and changing negative thought patterns and behaviors that contribute to distress. CBT empowers individuals to challenge their negative beliefs, develop healthier coping mechanisms, and improve their overall quality of life.

Group therapy can be particularly beneficial for men over 60, as it provides an opportunity to connect with peers facing similar challenges. Sharing experiences, listening to others' perspectives, and offering support can foster a sense of belonging and reduce feelings of isolation.

Group therapy also allows men to learn from one another's successes and setbacks, providing valuable insights and encouragement.

In addition to traditional therapy, alternative counseling options can also be explored. Art therapy, music therapy, and mindfulness-based therapies have shown promising results in promoting mental well-being among older adults. These approaches provide creative outlets for expression, relaxation, and self-reflection.

When seeking professional help, it is important to find a therapist or counselor who specializes in men's mental health after 60. They will have the expertise and experience to understand the unique challenges faced by older men and tailor their approach accordingly. Referrals from trusted friends, family members, or healthcare providers can be a good starting point in finding the right professional.

Remember, seeking therapy or counseling is a proactive step towards maintaining good mental health. It is never too late to seek help and find support on your journey towards emotional well-being.

Chapter 7: Building a Supportive Community

The Power of Support: Establishing Meaningful Connections

In the journey of life, reaching the golden years is a milestone worth celebrating. However, this phase often brings about unique challenges, particularly in the realm of mental health. As men over 60, it is crucial to acknowledge and prioritize our mental well-being. This subchapter delves into the power of support and the significance of establishing meaningful connections to navigate the complexities of men's mental health after 60.

One of the most formidable aspects of this stage of life is the potential for isolation. Retirement, loss of loved ones, and physical limitations can all contribute to a sense of loneliness. However, it is essential to recognize that we are not alone in this journey. By actively seeking out support, whether through family, friends, or support groups, we can cultivate a strong network of individuals who understand and empathize with our experiences. These connections become a lifeline, offering comfort, guidance, and a sense of belonging.

Meaningful connections go beyond mere companionship; they provide a safe space for sharing thoughts, fears, and aspirations. Men over 60 often face unique mental health challenges, such as depression, anxiety, or grief. By establishing these connections, we can break free from the stigma surrounding mental health and open up about our struggles. Sharing our stories not only lightens the burden we carry but also allows others to offer support and insights based on their own experiences.

Moreover, these connections can lead to the discovery of new passions and interests. Engaging in activities and hobbies with like-minded individuals can rejuvenate our spirits and provide a sense of purpose. Whether it's joining a book club, volunteering for a cause we care about, or participating in group fitness classes, the possibilities for exploration and growth are endless. These shared experiences foster a sense of camaraderie, boosting our overall well-being and mental health.

The power of support extends beyond our personal relationships. Seeking professional help, such as therapists or counselors specializing in men's mental health after 60, can be transformative. These experts understand the unique challenges we face and can provide guidance and strategies for managing our mental well-being. They can help us unpack our emotions, develop coping mechanisms, and establish healthy routines that promote a positive mindset.

In conclusion, establishing meaningful connections and seeking support are vital steps in navigating the complexities of men's mental health after 60. By surrounding ourselves with understanding individuals, sharing our stories, and engaging in activities that bring us joy, we can dismantle the barriers that often hinder our emotional well-being. Remember, you are not alone on this journey. Embrace the power of support, and together we can navigate the golden years with resilience and strength.

Men's Groups and Support Networks: Finding Camaraderie

In the golden years of life, it is not uncommon for men over 60 to experience various mental health challenges. The transition into retirement, loss of loved ones, and physical changes can often lead to feelings of isolation, depression, and anxiety. However, it is important to remember that you are not alone in this journey. The power of camaraderie and the support of like-minded individuals can make a significant difference in your mental well-being.

One of the most effective ways to combat the challenges of mental health after 60 is to seek out men's groups and support networks. These groups provide a safe and inclusive space for men to share their experiences, challenges, and triumphs. They offer a sense of belonging and understanding that can be difficult to find elsewhere.

Men's groups and support networks are designed to foster camaraderie among individuals who have walked similar paths in life. Whether you are a retiree adjusting to a new routine or a widower navigating life without a partner, these groups can provide a support system that understands your unique struggles. They offer a non-judgmental environment where you can freely express your emotions, fears, and hopes.

By engaging in group discussions, you gain valuable insights from others who have faced similar challenges. The wisdom and experiences shared within these groups can provide you with new perspectives, coping strategies, and a renewed sense of purpose. Moreover, the friendships formed in these networks often extend beyond the meeting room, leading to lasting bonds and social activities that enhance your overall well-being.

Joining a men's group or support network also offers a chance to explore new hobbies, interests, and passions. These groups often organize various activities such as hiking, golfing, book clubs, or volunteer work. Engaging in such activities not only helps you stay active and maintain a healthy lifestyle but also provides opportunities to connect with others who share similar interests.

In conclusion, navigating the challenges of men's mental health after 60 requires finding camaraderie and support. Men's groups and support networks offer a valuable platform for men over 60 to connect with like-minded individuals, share their experiences, and find solace in knowing they are not alone. By embracing the power of camaraderie, you can navigate the golden years with a renewed sense of purpose, emotional well-being, and a vibrant social life.

Communicating with Loved Ones: Strengthening Relationships

As men enter their golden years, it becomes increasingly important to prioritize mental health and nurture relationships with loved ones. This subchapter aims to provide guidance on how to effectively communicate with those closest to you, thereby strengthening bonds and promoting overall well-being.

One of the key aspects of maintaining healthy relationships is open and honest communication. Many men over 60 may have grown up in a time when discussing emotions was not encouraged, leading to potential barriers in communication. However, it is essential to break these barriers and express oneself genuinely. Sharing feelings, concerns, and joys with loved ones can create deeper connections and foster emotional support networks.

Active listening is another crucial component of effective communication. Taking the time to truly hear and understand what others are saying demonstrates respect and empathy. Engaging in meaningful conversations, asking open-ended questions, and acknowledging the thoughts and feelings of loved ones can help build stronger bonds and promote mutual understanding.

It is also important to remember that communication is a two-way street. While expressing oneself is vital, it is equally essential to listen and validate the thoughts and feelings of others. Showing empathy and being non-judgmental can create a safe space for loved ones to share their own emotions and concerns.

Technology has revolutionized the way we communicate, and embracing it can enhance relationships, especially in today's digital age.

Regularly connecting with loved ones through video calls, emails, or social media platforms can help bridge geographical distances and maintain a sense of closeness. Additionally, technology can provide opportunities for shared activities such as online games, virtual book clubs, or even just sending funny memes, fostering a sense of togetherness despite physical separation.

Lastly, it is crucial to make time for face-to-face interactions. While technology can be beneficial, nothing can replace the warmth and connection that comes from spending quality time with loved ones in person. Whether it's sharing a meal, going for walks, or participating in hobbies together, these shared experiences can strengthen relationships and create lasting memories.

In conclusion, effective communication is vital for men over 60 to maintain healthy relationships and promote mental well-being. By breaking down communication barriers, actively listening, embracing technology, and making time for face-to-face interactions, men can strengthen bonds with loved ones and navigate their golden years with a sense of fulfillment and happiness. Remember, it is never too late to invest in your relationships and prioritize your mental health.

Mentoring and Giving Back: Sharing Wisdom and Experience

As men entering the golden years, we have a wealth of wisdom and experience to offer to the world. Mentoring and giving back not only benefits others but also brings a sense of purpose and fulfillment to our own lives. In this subchapter, we will explore the importance of sharing our knowledge and how it can positively impact our mental health after 60.

One of the greatest gifts we can give is our time and support to others who may be going through similar challenges. By becoming mentors, we can provide guidance and encouragement to younger generations, helping them navigate the complexities of life. Whether it's mentoring a colleague at work, a neighbor, or even a grandchild, our experiences can offer valuable insights and lessons learned.

By engaging in mentoring relationships, we also foster a sense of connection and community, which is essential for maintaining good mental health. Loneliness and isolation can become more prevalent as we age, but by reaching out and sharing our wisdom, we can combat these feelings and create meaningful relationships.

Another way to give back is by volunteering our time and skills. There are countless organizations and causes that can benefit from our expertise and knowledge. Whether it's teaching a class, offering professional advice, or simply lending a helping hand, our contributions can make a significant difference in the lives of others. Not only does this provide a sense of purpose and fulfillment, but it also helps us stay mentally active and engaged.

Additionally, mentoring and giving back can be a powerful tool for personal growth and self-reflection. Sharing our experiences with others allows us to gain new perspectives and insights, further enriching our own lives. By actively engaging in mentoring relationships, we continue to learn and grow, challenging ourselves to constantly improve and adapt.

In conclusion, mentoring and giving back plays a crucial role in men's mental health after 60. By sharing our wisdom and experience with others, we not only contribute to the betterment of society but also find purpose, connection, and personal growth. Let us embrace the opportunity to mentor and give back, for it is through these acts that we can truly navigate and thrive in our golden years.

Chapter 8: Embracing Aging with Resilience and Positivity

Embracing Age-Related Changes: Accepting and Adapting

As men enter their golden years, it is not uncommon to face various age-related changes that can impact their mental health. However, it is essential to understand that embracing these changes and adapting to them can lead to a more fulfilling and satisfying life. In this subchapter, we will explore the importance of accepting and adapting to age-related changes, and how it can positively impact men's mental health after 60.

Accepting age-related changes is the first step towards maintaining good mental health. It is natural for men to experience physical changes such as decreased energy levels, changes in sleep patterns, or even a decline in sexual function. These changes can be frustrating and may lead to feelings of inadequacy or loss of identity. By accepting these changes as a part of the aging process, men can focus on finding alternative ways to maintain their overall well-being.

Adapting to age-related changes is crucial for men to thrive in their golden years. This may involve making adjustments to daily routines, such as incorporating regular exercise tailored to their abilities or modifying their diet to support optimal health. Adapting also means seeking support from healthcare professionals who can provide guidance on managing age-related conditions and ensuring that mental health is prioritized.

Furthermore, adapting to age-related changes requires men to embrace new roles and find a sense of purpose beyond their previous careers. Retirement can be a significant life transition, and it is important to explore new hobbies, interests, or even volunteering opportunities that bring joy and fulfillment. Engaging in social activities and maintaining strong connections with loved ones can also contribute to improved mental well-being.

Navigating age-related changes may also involve addressing any underlying mental health issues. Depression and anxiety can be more prevalent in older men, and seeking professional help to manage these conditions is vital. Men over 60 should understand that mental health concerns are common and should not be stigmatized or ignored.

In conclusion, embracing age-related changes and adapting to them is a fundamental aspect of men's mental health after 60. Accepting these changes allows men to focus on maintaining overall well-being, while adapting to new circumstances and roles can lead to a more fulfilling life. By prioritizing mental health, seeking support, and addressing any underlying concerns, men can navigate their golden years with confidence, resilience, and a renewed sense of purpose.

Positive Aging: Challenging Ageist Stereotypes and Beliefs

As men enter their golden years, they often find themselves bombarded with negative stereotypes and beliefs about aging. These ageist views can have a detrimental impact on their mental health and overall well-being. However, it is important to recognize that positive aging is not only possible but also essential for men over 60.

Society often portrays older adults as frail, forgetful, and disconnected from the world around them. These stereotypes can lead to a sense of self-doubt and a loss of identity for men entering this phase of life. However, it is crucial to challenge these ageist beliefs and embrace the opportunities that come with aging.

One key aspect of positive aging is maintaining good mental health. Many men over 60 may face unique challenges in this area, such as retirement, loss of loved ones, or health issues. However, it is important to remember that mental health is just as important as physical health. Engaging in activities that promote mental well-being, such as socializing, staying physically active, and pursuing hobbies, can greatly enhance one's overall quality of life.

Another important factor in positive aging is fostering meaningful connections and relationships. Men over 60 often find themselves at a crossroads, with children grown and careers winding down. However, this is an opportunity to cultivate new relationships, whether it be through joining community groups, volunteering, or reconnecting with old friends. Building a support network can provide a sense of belonging and purpose, combating feelings of isolation and loneliness.

Furthermore, positive aging involves embracing one's wisdom and experience. Men over 60 have a wealth of knowledge and life lessons to share. Engaging in activities that allow for self-reflection, such as journaling or mentoring younger individuals, can help men appreciate their unique perspectives and contributions to society.

In conclusion, positive aging is about challenging ageist stereotypes and beliefs that hinder men's mental health after 60. By focusing on mental well-being, fostering meaningful connections, and embracing life experiences, men can navigate their golden years with a sense of purpose, fulfillment, and joy. It is never too late to rewrite the narrative and embrace the incredible potential for growth and happiness that comes with aging.

Celebrating Life's Milestones: Finding Joy in the Golden Years

Subchapter: Celebrating Life's Milestones: Finding Joy in the Golden Years

Introduction:

Life is a journey filled with various milestones, and reaching the golden years is undoubtedly one of the most significant achievements. As men over 60, you have experienced a multitude of challenges and triumphs, shaping you into the individuals you are today. This subchapter will explore the importance of celebrating life's milestones and finding joy in the golden years, with a specific focus on men's mental health after 60.

Embracing Milestones:

As you enter this new phase of life, it is crucial to embrace and celebrate the milestones you have achieved. Reflect on the challenges you have overcome, the lessons you have learned, and the wisdom you have gained. Recognize that each milestone is a testament to your resilience, strength, and character. By acknowledging these achievements, you can boost your self-esteem and cultivate a positive outlook on life.

The Power of Perspective:

Finding joy in the golden years often lies in the power of perspective. It is natural for life to present its fair share of ups and downs, but how we perceive and respond to these events can significantly impact our mental health. By adopting a positive mindset and reframing negative experiences, you can find joy even in the face of adversity. Celebrating life's milestones becomes a way of appreciating the journey rather than solely focusing on the destination.

Creating Meaningful Connections:

Another essential aspect of finding joy in the golden years is through the fostering of meaningful connections. Surrounding yourself with loved ones, friends, and a supportive community can have a profound impact on your mental well-being. Celebrating milestones together allows for shared joy and reinforces the importance of human connection. Engaging in activities that bring you closer to others, such as joining clubs or volunteering, can provide a sense of purpose and fulfillment.

Maintaining Physical and Mental Well-being:

To fully enjoy life's milestones, it is essential to prioritize your physical and mental well-being. Engage in regular exercise, maintain a balanced diet, and ensure you get enough restorative sleep. Additionally, taking care of your mental health is equally important. Consider incorporating mindfulness or meditation practices into your routine, seeking therapy if needed, and exploring new hobbies or interests that bring you joy.

Conclusion:

The golden years are a time to celebrate the milestones you have achieved and find joy in the present moment. By embracing your accomplishments, adopting a positive mindset, fostering meaningful connections, and prioritizing your physical and mental well-being, you can navigate this phase of life with grace and fulfillment. Celebrate each milestone as a testament to your strength and resilience, and let the golden years be a time of joy, growth, and appreciation for all that life has to offer.

Leaving a Legacy: Reflecting on Your Life's Journey

As men over 60, we have experienced a lifetime of trials, triumphs, and everything in between. Now, in the golden years of our lives, it is an opportune time to reflect on our life's journey and consider the legacy we want to leave behind. This subchapter will delve into the importance of reflecting on our past, identifying our values, and finding meaning in our lives.

Reflecting on our life's journey allows us to gain a deeper understanding of ourselves and the experiences that have shaped us. It is an opportunity to celebrate our achievements, acknowledge our mistakes, and make peace with our past. By taking the time to reflect, we can gain valuable insights, wisdom, and closure that will contribute to our mental well-being.

Identifying our values is an integral part of leaving a meaningful legacy. What are the principles that have guided us throughout our lives? What are the beliefs and ideals we hold dear? By aligning our actions with our values, we can ensure that our legacy reflects our core essence. It is never too late to reassess our priorities and make changes that will bring us closer to living a life in harmony with our values.

In conclusion, reflecting on our life's journey, identifying our values, and finding meaning are crucial aspects of leaving a legacy as men over 60. By doing so, we can ensure that our golden years are filled with purpose, fulfillment, and mental well-being. Let us embark on this journey together and make our mark on the world, leaving a legacy that generations to come will remember.

Conclusion: Navigating Your Golden Years with Confidence and Mental Well-being

Finding meaning in our lives becomes increasingly important as we age. It is through the pursuit of purpose and passion that we can make the most of our golden years. This subchapter will explore different avenues for finding meaning, such as engaging in hobbies, volunteering, mentoring, or pursuing new interests. By actively seeking out opportunities to make a difference, we can leave a lasting legacy that extends beyond our own lives.

Navigating the golden years can be a complex journey, but taking the time to reflect on our life's journey, identify our values, and find meaning will contribute to our mental health and overall well-being. By consciously leaving a legacy that aligns with our values and passions, we can feel a sense of fulfillment and purpose in this new chapter of our lives.

As we conclude this guide on men's mental health after 60, it is important to acknowledge the unique challenges and opportunities that come with navigating your golden years. This stage of life presents a significant transition, both physically and emotionally, and it is crucial to prioritize your mental well-being during this time.

One of the key takeaways from this book is the importance of seeking support and maintaining social connections. Loneliness and isolation can have detrimental effects on mental health, so it is essential to actively engage in social activities and nurture relationships with family and friends. Remember, you are not alone in this journey, and there are resources available to help you through any difficulties you may encounter.

Another significant aspect of maintaining mental well-being is taking care of your physical health. Engaging in regular exercise, eating a balanced diet, and getting enough sleep are all crucial for overall well-being. Physical activity not only helps to keep your body fit but also has positive effects on your mental health, reducing symptoms of anxiety and depression. Additionally, a healthy diet can provide essential nutrients that support brain health and cognitive function.

It is also important to prioritize self-care and engage in activities that bring you joy and fulfillment. This could involve pursuing hobbies, spending time in nature, or practicing relaxation techniques such as meditation or deep breathing exercises. Taking time for yourself and doing things that make you happy can greatly contribute to your mental well-being and overall satisfaction in life.

Lastly, it is crucial to be aware of the signs of mental health issues and seek professional help if needed. Mental health conditions do not discriminate based on age, and it is important to address any concerns or symptoms that may arise. Whether it is through therapy, counseling, or support groups, there are resources available specifically tailored to men over 60.

Remember, your mental well-being is just as important as your physical health. By prioritizing your mental well-being, seeking support, maintaining social connections, taking care of your physical health, engaging in self-care, and being aware of mental health issues, you can navigate your golden years with confidence and enjoy a fulfilling and satisfying life.

In conclusion, this guide has provided valuable insights and strategies to help men over 60 navigate their golden years with confidence and mental well-being. Remember, you are not alone, and there are resources available to support you on this journey. Embrace this stage of life with a positive mindset, take care of yourself, and live your best life in your golden years.